Treat Your Own Iliotibial Band Syndrome

by
Jim Johnson, PT

Drawings by Eunice Johnson
© 2013 Jim Johnson
All Rights Reserved.

First published by Dog Ear Publishing
4010 W. 86th Street, Ste H
Indianapolis, IN 46268
www.dogearpublishing.net

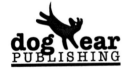

ISBN: 978-1-4575-1760-0
Library of Congress Control Number: 2013902628

This paper is acid free paper.
Printed in the United States of America

How This Book Is Set Up

✓ Learn what the iliotibial band is and where it's at in *Chapter 1*.

✓ Find out what causes iliotibial band syndrome in *Chapter 2*.

✓ Learn how to get rid of the inflammation in your knee in *Chapter 3*.

✓ Learn how to strengthen your hip abductors and why it's so important in *Chapter 4*.

✓ Find out how to correctly stretch the iliotibial band in *Chapter 5*.

✓ Get started on the 6-week rehabilitation program in *Chapter 6*.

✓ Monitor your progress with the tools in *Chapter 7*.

Why Is The Print In This Book So Big?

People who read my books sometimes wonder why the print is so big in many of them. Some tend to think it's because I'm trying to make a little book bigger or a short book longer.

Actually, the main reason I use bigger print is for the same reason I intentionally write short books, usually under 100 pages–it's just plain easier to read and get the information quicker!

You see, the books I write address common, everyday problems that people of *all* ages have. In other words, the "typical" reader of my books could be a teenager, a busy housewife, a CEO, a construction worker, or a retired senior citizen with poor eyesight. Therefore, by writing books with larger print that are short and to the point, *everyone* can get the information quickly and with ease. After all, what good is a book full of useful information if nobody ever finishes it?

Table of Contents

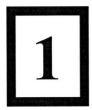

Iliotibial Band Syndrome - So What Exactly Is *That*?

To answer that question, of course it helps to know what the iliotibial band actually is.

To begin with, it's pronounced *ill-ee-o-tibb-ee-ull* band. The word iliotibial itself is made up from a combination of the words *ilium* and *tibia* - which are two bones you have in your hip and leg...

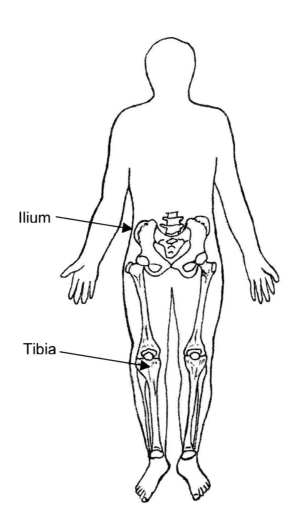

Figure 1. The ilium and tibia bones.

And someone picked these particular two bones because they're the ones that mark the beginning and end of where a tough band of tissue lies – hence the term *iliotibial band*.

In the picture below, the arrow points to the iliotibial band, and the dotted line shows us it's path as it runs up and down the side of your leg – all the way from the ilium bone, down to the tibia bone…

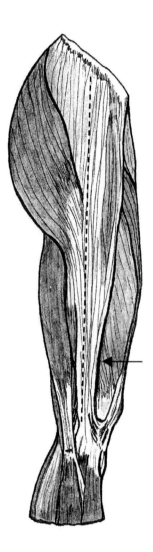

Figure 1. The right leg from the side – the iliotibial band and its path

And here's a few more pictures of how it looks from different angles – the arrows once again pointing to the iliotibial band. As you can see, the iliotibial band runs mainly down *the side* of your leg, and doesn't extend very far to the front or back...

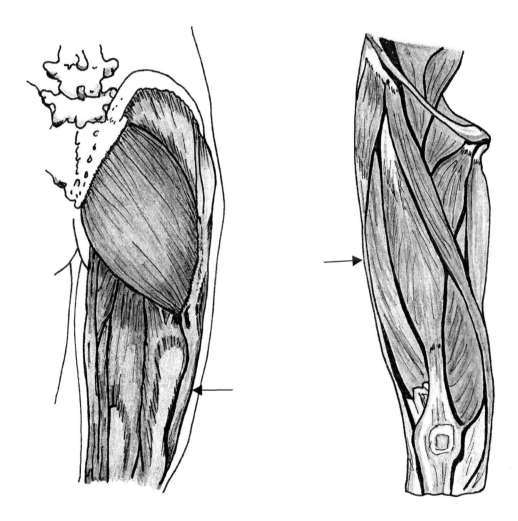

Figures 2 and 3. Views of the iliotibial band as it's seen from the back and front of the right leg.

It does get a little more interesting around the knee, however, where the iliotibial band inserts into the tibia…

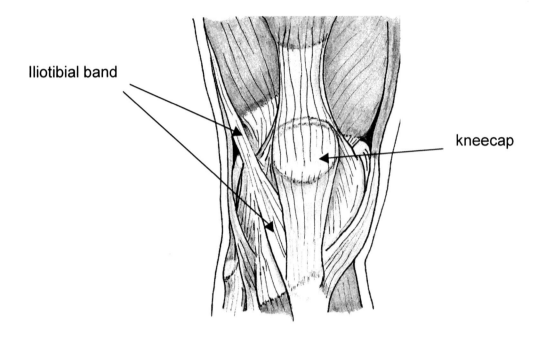

Figure 4. The right front knee – close-up of where the iliotibial band inserts.

So What's It Made Of?

Good question. Since you know where the iliotibial band is, and have an idea of what it looks like, what the heck is the thing made of? Is it a muscle? A ligament?

Well, the iliotibial band actually consists of a specialized tissue known as *fascia*. Fascia is a type of connective tissue that can be found everywhere in your body. Made up of *collagen* and *elastin* fibers, there's a layer of this fascia stuff right under your skin, around your organs, and for that matter, even around each of your muscles! Best thought of as a kind of "packing material," one of the big jobs of fascia is to provide support to the many different structures throughout your body.

Not all fascia is created equal however. For example, some of the fascia in your body is laid out much like a thin sheet of tissue paper. If you've ever removed the skin from a chicken breast, that white film-like substance right underneath the skin you may have noticed was actually a very thin layer of fascia – which is quite similar to how it looks in humans too.

The fascia that makes up your iliotibial band, on the other hand, is not nearly this thin. In fact, it's one of the thickest and strongest pieces of fascia in the entire human body! As such, it helps to stabilize your knee and provides a place for many of your muscles to attach to.

Finding Your Iliotibial Band

Okay, you've seen a lot of drawings of the iliotibial band, now its time to find it on yourself. Sound hard? Not really. All you have to do is sit in a chair and raise you knee up. When your foot lifts up off the floor, whallah, the iliotibial band jumps into action and stands right out!

The arrow in the picture below points to the lower part of the iliotibial band as it is heading in a straight line right to the knee. Try rubbing your finger over it like you're strumming a guitar – pretty tough stuff that fascia...

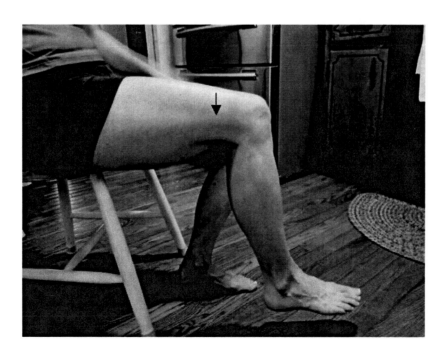

So What Exactly Is Iliotibial Band Syndrome?

Now that you're more familiar with your iliotibial band, or should I say bands, since you have one on each side, we can talk about what iliotibial band syndrome is.

In short, iliotibial band syndrome is when you have an inflamed area *under* the iliotibial band where it passes along the side of your knee. The drawing below shows us the consistent spot where iliotibial band syndrome occurs...

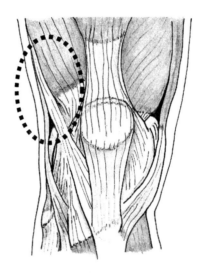

Figure 5. Looking at the right knee from the front. Circle shows
the main area of pain in iliotibial band syndrome.

Here's a list of some of the most common symptoms people get when they have iliotibial band syndrome:

- they get a sharp pain or burning on the side of their knee - which can also radiate up or down

- activities that require repetitive knee bending, especially at around a 30 degree angle, cause pain

- going up or down stairs is often times painful

- runners commonly report starting out pain free, but then develop pain after a predictable time or distance. Downhill running can particularly aggravate things.

- early on in the iliotibial band syndrome, symptoms can subside shortly after a run, but then return with the next run. As the problem progresses, pain can persist even with walking.

- sitting for long periods of time with the knee bent causes pain, while keeping the knee straight feels better

As you can see from this list of commonly reported symptoms, it's the over and over knee bending that seems to cause the most pain when you have iliotibial band syndrome. But why is that?

Key Points

✓ the iliotibial band is made up of a connective tissue known as *fascia*

✓ it's called the iliotibial band because the band runs from the ilium bone, down to the tibia bone – hence the term "iliotibial"

✓ iliotibial band syndrome is when you have an inflamed area *under* the iliotibial band where it passes over the side of your knee.

✓ the most common site of pain in iliotibial band syndrome is on the side of the knee.

✓ activities that cause the knee to bend over and over, particularly at a 30 degree angle, typically cause the most pain

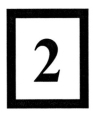 How Did I Get Iliotibial Band Syndrome?

I can tell you how you most likely got iliotibial band syndrome in one word: overuse. The story goes something like this.

First, know that as you use your legs throughout the day, you're contracting the muscles that make them move, which in turn are pulling hard on your tendons and other things they are connected to, like your iliotibial band. And, just like most things in your body, all these structures need time (at some point) to rest and repair themselves from this normal daily wear and tear. Not to mention the fact that if you exercise a lot, as with running, they need even more time to recover.

Therefore, if you work and stress your body's structures (like the muscles or iliotibial band), and give them *enough* time to recover each day, they're going to stay in good shape. We could then say that your body's structures are "keeping up" with your activities. And all is well.

Now let's say you have a day where you've worked your legs *more* than normal, or you're just using them in a way they're simply not used to. For example, maybe you were on your feet a lot more at work, or decided to double your running distance. Well, of course this is going to cause *more* wear and tear than your legs are normally used to, right?

Well, here's where the problems can start. **If** you give your legs time to rest and recover (meaning that they have time to make the necessary repairs from this increased stress) *before* using them a lot again, your body will be able to "keep up", and stay in good working order.

On the other hand, let's say you *continue* to repeatedly work your legs harder than usual and they don't get enough time off to recover and make repairs. What will happen to them then? Well, *over time* areas of your legs (like the side of your knee where the iliotibial band passes) might not be able to "keep up" with the activities you ask them to do, and will eventually run into problems.

The moral of the story? The main cause of iliotibial band syndrome in the majority of cases is one of **overuse,** because your body was repeatedly put through stressful activities – and then not given enough repair time. Overworked areas then respond by becoming inflamed. Oddly enough, however, while we've named this problem iliotibial band syndrome, the iliotibial band isn't the structure that gets inflamed…

So Where Exactly Is The Problem At?

We know that the main area of pain when you have iliotibial band syndrome is on the *side* of the knee. Further investigation also tells us that that's the spot where most patients are the most tender too – right over their iliotibial band. So it makes sense then, that you have an inflamed iliotibial band, right?

Not exactly. Approaching this matter scientifically, as we do everything in this book, to say that something is "inflamed" means that we should be able to find some hard evidence of inflammation. Without getting too caught up in details, inflammation can be broken down into two general patterns, *acute* and *chronic*. Here's the difference between the two:

- *acute inflammation* is an immediate and early response to tissue injury. It comes on quickly, but lasts for minutes, hours, or a few days. Neutrophils are the major kind of cells that are involved in acute inflammation.

- *chronic inflammation* is inflammation of a prolonged duration, such as weeks or months. Some of the major types of cells that are involved in chronic inflammation include macrophages, lymphocytes, and plasma cells.

Now it's *not* important to know all about the different types of cells, although you may be interested to know that a lot of them are simply different types of white blood cells. What is important, however, is to know that these are exactly the kinds of cells we should be able to find in the iliotibial band *if* it is indeed "inflamed" – since these are the cells directly involved in the body's inflammatory process.

Well, let's see what the surgeons have found when they've cut open the knees of patients with iliotibial band syndrome and examined the tissue under a microscope...

- in this study, 21 patients with chronic iliotibial band syndrome were operated on (Nemeth 1996)

- samples were taken of the tissue *under* the iliotibial band and looked at under a microscope

- the biopsy results revealed chronic inflammation, hyperplasia, fibrosis, and mucoid degeneration

- another study looked at 100 patients with iliotibial band syndrome (Noble 1980). All of them were runners.

- 5 patients ended up having surgery

- samples of the tissue taken *under* the iliotibial band at surgery revealed inflammatory cells

That's interesting, don't you think? The studies seem to be reporting inflammation, but the inflamed area is *under* the iliotibial band, not in the iliotibial band itself.

While you just won't find a lot of studies on iliotibial band syndrome that have examined tissue samples taken at surgery (the iliotibial band syndrome is not a highly researched subject), what research has been done in this area all consistently points to the same thing – inflammation *under* the iliotibial band. Having said that, I wonder what we'd find if we looked at people with iliotibial band syndrome with an MRI...

- 6 patients with iliotibial band syndrome were examined with MRI (Murphy 1992). Results showed abnormal signals *deep* to the iliotibial band consistent with fluid collection and swelling. No abnormalities were seen in the iliotibial band itself.

- 16 cases of iliotibial band syndrome were investigated with MRI (Muhle 1999). Researchers found abnormal signals and fluid collections *deep* to the iliotibial band. The iliotibial band was normal.

- 4 patients with iliotibial band syndrome had MRI's of their knees (Nishimura 1997). Findings revealed inflammation and/or swelling *under* the iliotibial band. No abnormalities were found in the iliotibial band itself.

Seems the MRI scanner is finding the same thing the surgeons are: an area of inflammation *under* a normal iliotibial band. But how did the inflammation end up in that spot?

Friction or Compression?

So if you've got inflammation in a spot, it's usually because there's something irritating the area. In the case of iliotibial band syndrome, the most popular theory is that it's the iliotibial band rubbing over your knee bone that causes the inflammation and pain. Here's how that works…

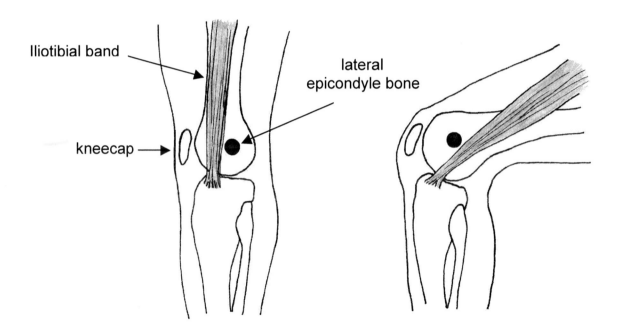

Iliotibial band

lateral epicondyle bone

kneecap

Figure 6. Looking at the left knee from the side. Note that the when the knee is straight, the iliotibial band lies **in front** of the dot. The dot represents a part of your knee bone that sticks out, called the lateral epicondyle.

Figure 7. As you bend your knee, note how the iliotibial band has now passed *over* the dot (the bony lateral epicondyle that sticks out) and is now **behind** it. The theory is that this repetitive rubbing of the iliotibial band *over* the bony lateral epicondyle is what creates the inflammation and pain.

So as you can see, the main idea here, is that as your knee bends back and forth, for example with running, the iliotibial band rubs over a part of the knee bone that sticks out – thus creating inflammation and pain.

You have to admit, it does make a lot of sense, and this has been the major theory for years – in fact that's why you've probably heard of iliotibial band *friction* syndrome.

However I'm not so sure that's what's really going on. Why? Because if you dig around in the iliotibial band research, there's a lot of evidence that tells me that the problem is created not by friction, but rather by *compression*. Let me explain. The first big problem with the idea that the iliotibial band rubs over the lateral epicondyle, is the fact that the iliotibial band itself is not an isolated structure, but rather it's just a thickened, *continuous* part of the fascia that envelopes your whole thigh. Here's a drawing that illustrates this…

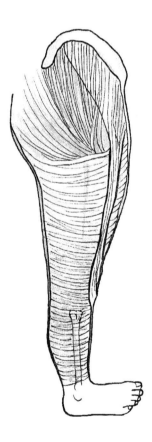

Figure 8. The fascia of the right leg. Just under the skin lies a sheet of fascia that winds around and envelops the leg. Your iliotibial band is just a thickened part of this circumferential fascia – it runs continuous with it, not separate from it.

So because the iliotibial band is just a thickened part of the whole fascia that winds horizontally around your leg, it would be really hard to visualize how it could move back and forth.

I admit, while I have examined thin patients, the iliotibial band does indeed look like it moves over the lateral epicondyle as the knee bends. However closer inspection shows that this is not the case. What actually is happening, rather, is that the iliotibial band is put under tension from its front edge to its back edge as the knee bends – which only gives the illusion that it actually is moving from front to back.

And the research confirms this. In an interesting study (Fairclough 2006), researchers took MRI pictures of subjects as they moved their knees. And what do you think they saw the iliotibial band do? Well, as subjects bent their knee, the iliotibial band was seen to actually be *compressed* into the bony side of the knee, not rubbing over it!

Apparently iliotibial band syndrome is not a problem with the iliotibial band rubbing over a bone – it's a problem with the iliotibial band repetitively *compressing into* the side of the knee – and irritating the tissue underneath. And remember - this is exactly what the tissue samples have found – a normal iliotibial band with inflamed tissue underneath.

Further adding to the compression theory, is the fact that there are several anatomical studies that have dissected the knee and found the iliotibial band to be firmly anchored along the length of your entire leg bone by fibrous strands – making it hard for it to slide back and forth (Fairclough 2006 and Falvey 2010).

Okay, now that we have a better understanding of the problems that are actually going on in your knee, we can treat those problems accordingly. First up, let's treat that inflammation under the iliotibial band...

Key Points

✓ in the majority of cases, iliotibial band syndrome is caused by oversuse

✓ tissue samples taken from people who have iliotibial band syndrome show that there is inflammation *under* the iliotibial band

✓ interestingly, MRI studies done on people with iliotibial band syndrome show the iliotibial band itself to be quite normal

✓ there is little evidence to support the theory that the inflamed area under the iliotibial band is caused by friction

✓ it is much more likely that the area under the iliotibial band becomes inflamed by the iliotibial band repeatedly *compressing* that area

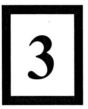

How to Get Rid of the Inflammation

So we know from the surgical tissue samples that there's an inflamed spot under the iliotibial band that's causing all the pain. One way to treat it would be to get a cortisone shot into the area. For instance a randomized controlled trial done on runners showed that that it effectively decreased pain during running (Gunter 2003).

However not everybody is crazy about being stuck with needles, and since this book is called "Treat Your Own Iliotibial Band Syndrome", we need to talk about what can you do yourself to get rid of the inflammation. And probably the best tool I have is called *ice massage*.

Now most people know that ice is good to get down swelling, but it's actually a much more powerful tool than you might realize. A quick look at the research tells us there's some big advantages to using ice massage...

- a five minute ice massage can cause a drop in temperature of 18° C and reach a depth of at least 2 centimeters (Lowden 1975)

- ice massage has been shown to decrease skin and muscle temperatures much quicker than an ice pack (Zemke 1998)

In short, ice massage can drop the temperature under your skin fast! Furthermore, it's very inexpensive to do and takes very little time. Here's how you do it...

You'll need three things: a styrofoam cup, plain tap water, and a freezer. Start by getting the styrofoam cup out…

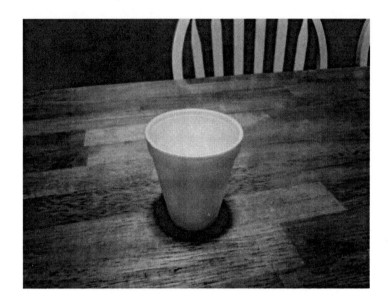

Now go to the sink and fill the cup up about ¾ of the way full…

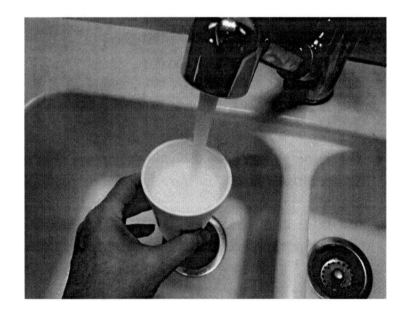

Now carefully put the cup in the freezer…

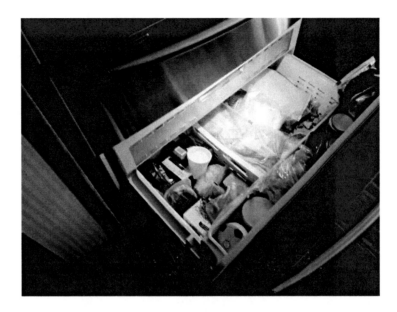

When the water has frozen and turned into ice, take it out of the freezer. Then turn the cup upside down and start peeling away the styrofoam. As you peel away *the bottom* of the cup, it will begin to look like this...

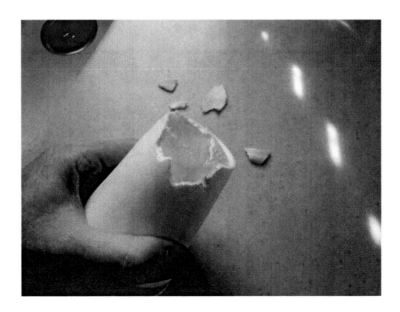

Whoo-hoo – we're almost there! Continue to peel away the styrofoam until it looks something like this…

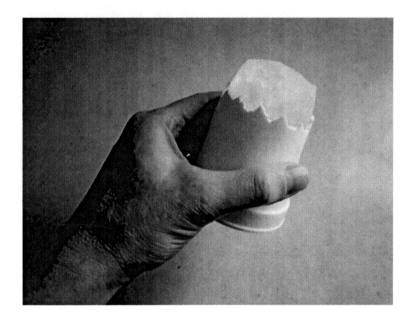

With your newly made anti-inflammation tool in hand, find that painful tender area on the side of your knee. Using small circular motions, massage the area with the ice. It should be looking something like this…

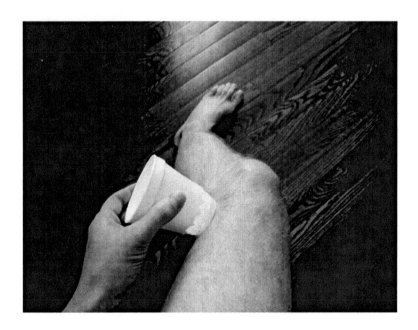

How long do you massage the ice into the painful, tender area? Based on the studies at the beginning of this chapter, I recommend about five minutes. If you can't hold out that long, its good to know that tissue temperature starts to drop significantly within a minute or two of ice massage, so just do it as long as you can – with five minutes being the max. As usual, it's always a good idea to check with your doctor before doing ice massage just in case you have a medical condition that prohibits you from using ice.

Key Points

✓ **ice massage is an easy way to decrease inflammation right where you need to**

✓ **a five minute ice massage can cause a drop in temperature of 18° C and reach a depth of at least 2 centimeters**

✓ **ice massage has been shown to decrease skin and muscle temperatures much quicker than an ice pack**

✓ **freezing a styrofoam cup filled with water is a cheap, convenient way to perform ice massage**

Strengthen Your Hip Abductors

What's a hip abductor? And what's something at the hip have to do with pain at your knee? Well, let's start with…

Hip Abduction

Abduction is a motion – more specifically, it's when you're moving a body part *away* from your midline. Hip abduction, then, is when you're moving your leg away from your body, out to the side. A picture is worth a thousand words, soooo….

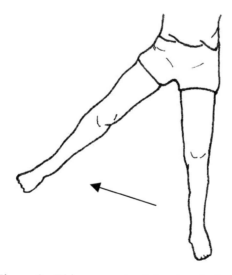

Figure 9. This person is abducting their right leg.

And it makes no difference if you 're standing or lying, if you're moving your leg out to the side, well, it's still hip abduction…

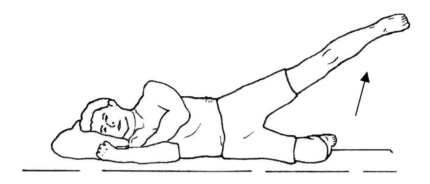

Figure 10. This person is abducting their left leg.

So now you know what hip abduction is. The next thing you need to know is that there's a little muscle in your hip that is key in helping you perform this motion. It's known as the *gluteus medius*. Here's a picture of where it's at and what it looks like…

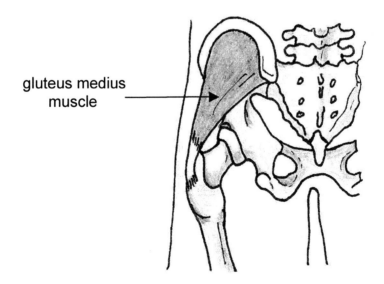

gluteus medius muscle

Figure 11. Looking at the right hip from the front – the gluteus medius.

While the gluteus medius is a relatively small muscle, it can cause some *big* problems if it's weak. Because it attaches to your pelvis as well as your leg bone, it also has the job of keeping your hips and pelvis level as you walk.

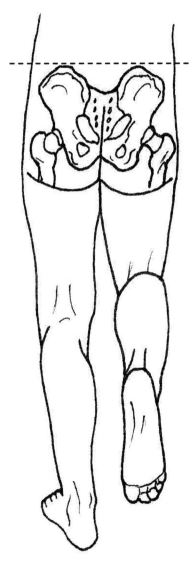 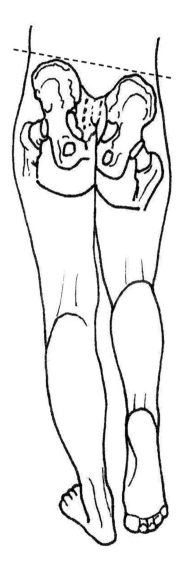

Figure 12. A strong gluteus medius helps keeps the pelvis level as you walk or run.

Figure 13. A weak gluteus medius can cause the pelvis to tilt as you walk. In this case, the right hip drops because the *left* gluteus medius is weak and can't hold it up.

The point to all this is not to give you a biomechanics lesson, but to let you know that a weakness in a muscle way up at the hip, *can* cause alignment problems and definitely make trouble for your knee. Which is exactly what the research has found…

- this study looked at 24 distance runners with iliotibial band syndrome, and compared them to a control group of 30 injury-free runners (Fredericson 2000)

- both groups had the strength of their gluteus medius muscles tested

- researchers found that the runners with iliotibial band syndrome had a weaker gluteus medius in their injured leg compared to their non-injured leg

- runners with iliotibial band syndrome also had much weaker gluteus medius muscles in their injured leg compared to the control group of non-injured runners

- interestingly, after 6-weeks of doing gluteus medius strengthening exercises, 22 out of the 24 runners with iliotibial band syndrome were pain-free

- at 6-months follow-up, there were no reports of recurrences

This is not the only study that has found gluteus medius weakness in people with iliotibial band syndrome either. One study looking at overuse injuries in runners found that those with iliotibial band symdrome had weak gluteus medius muscles (Niemuth 2005). Yet another study also found weak gluteus medius muscles in patients with iliotibial band syndrome, and noted that as they strengthened this muscle, subjects improved (Beers 2008). I guess it's time now for me to show you how to strengthen your gluteus medius…

The Exercises

As you've just read, there's a lot of research showing us that strengthening your gluteus medius can really help people with iliotibial band syndrome. So without further delay, here are two exercises that come directly from the studies you've just been reading about...

Sidelying Abduction Exercise

Step 1

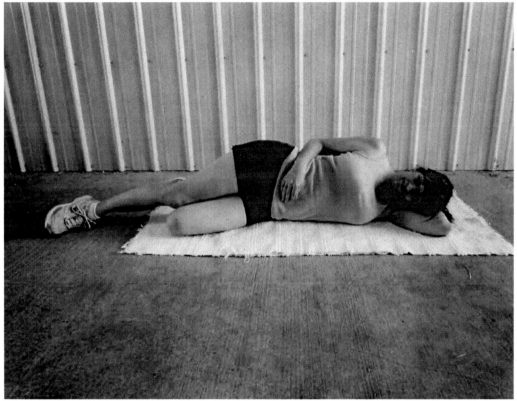

- find a comfortable place to lay down (the floor or on a bed will do)

- get into the above position – your painful knee should be on top

- in the above picture, the person is about to exercise the *right* gluteus medius

Step 2

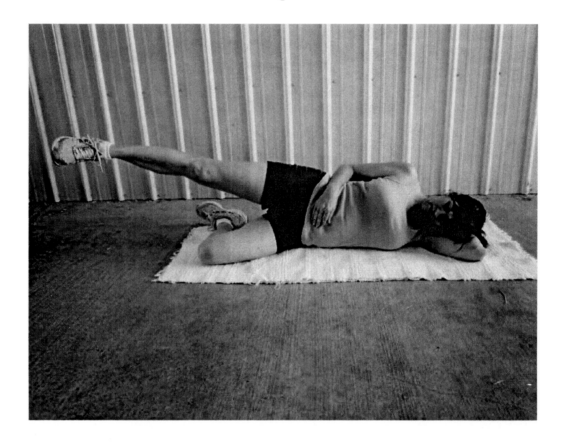

- now, keeping your knee straight, raise your leg straight up slowly. It should take you 3-4 seconds to raise your leg up.

- you don't need to go any higher than the picture shows

Step 3

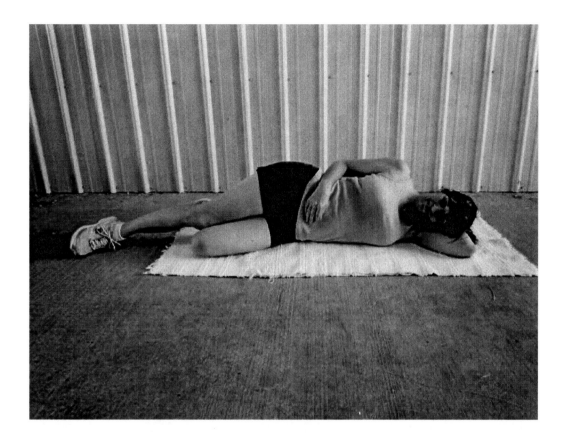

- return your leg to the starting position
- you've just done one repetiton
- repeat this for a total of 12 repetitions
- when you can do this 12 times in a row, add a one or two pound ankle weight to make the muscle stronger
- as you continue to add more weight over time, your gluteus medius will become stronger and stronger
- do this exercise one time a day, three times a week with a day of rest in between – for example Monday, Wednesday, Friday, or Tuesday, Thursday, Saturday

Hip Hike Exercise

Step 1

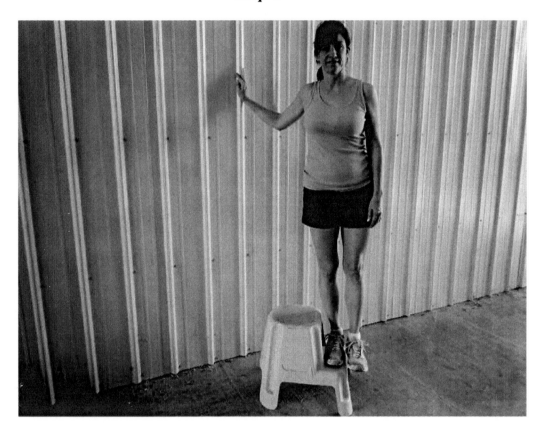

- get into the above position – a stair step or step stool will do
- your painful leg will be the one hanging off the step
- note that the foot hanging down MUST be level with the other foot
- make sure you have something to hold on to for balance

Step 2

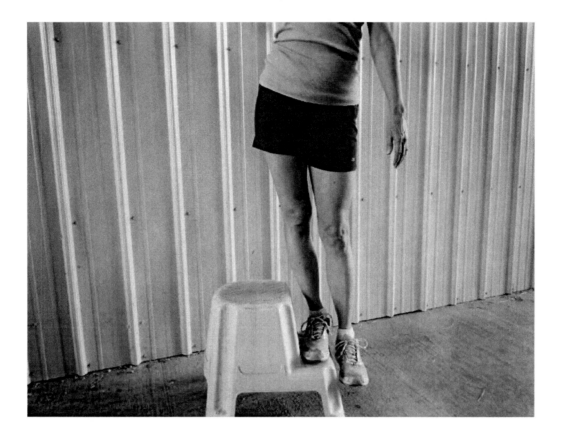

- keeping both legs straight *and next to each other,* slowly lower the foot of your painful leg down to the floor 4 or 5 inches as in the picture – this should take you 2-3 seconds. **Your knees stay straight – this motion comes from the hip.**

- you will have one foot and hip lower than the other at this point (remember, this is a gluteus medius exercise, and one job of the gluteus medius is to keep your hips level)

Step 3

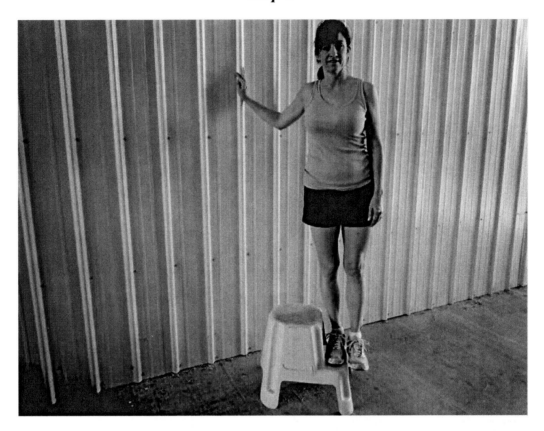

- now return your foot back up to the starting position so it is level with the other foot – your hips will be level now too.

- you've just done one repetiton

- repeat this for a total of 12 repetitions

- when you can do this 12 times in a row, add a one or two pound ankle weight to make the muscle stronger

- as you continue add more weight over time, your gluteus medius will become stronger and stronger

- do this exercise one time a day, three times a week with a day of rest in between – for example Monday, Wednesday, Friday, or Tuesday, Thursday, Saturday

- as you can see, this exercise is really just hiking your hip up and down, which gives the gluteus medius a good workout

Key Points

✓ the gluteus medius is an important muscle that moves your leg and keeps your pelvis lined up properly

✓ many studies have found that people with iliotibial band syndrome have weak gluteus medius muscles

✓ studies have also shown that when people with iliotibial band syndrome strengthen their abductors, they get better

✓ strengthening the gluteus medius muscle takes only a few minutes every other day

✓ always check with your doctor before beginning an exercise program

5 Stretch Your Iliotibial Band

Recall from Chapter 1 that the iliotibial band starts out at the hip, and ends at the knee:

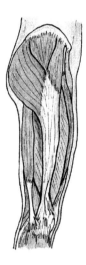

Looking at the above picture, it's not hard to visualize how a tight iliotibial band, whether the tightness be in the band itself or the muscles at the top that connect to it, could contribute to increased compression at the side of your knee where all the pain is. Several other factors also tell us that's its just a good idea for people with iliotibial band syndrome to be stretching...

- many studies have included stretching as part of a treatment program for iliotibial band syndrome and have gotten good results (Beers 2008, Fredericson 2000, Schwellnus 1991)

- some studies comparing people with iliotibial band syndrome to pain-free controls have found that those with iliotibial band syndrome have a decreased ability to *adduct* their hip (bring the legs together) - indicating tightness in the hip abductors (like the gluteus medius) or the iliotibial band (Grau 2011)

With all these reasons, taking the time to stretch your iliotibial band for a few minutes each day will be well worth the effort...

The Stretches

The pictures coming up represent a *series* of stretches – starting with a light, beginning stretch, and moving forward to more advanced, heavy-duty stretches. What you'll want to do is start with Stretch #1. If you feel a good stretch, stick with that one.

On the other hand, if the first stretch seems too easy, and you don't feel much of a stretch, try the next one until you find the one that stretches you out the best.

Having instructed hundreds of patients over the years in all kinds of stretches, I have learned that there is no one stretch that works for everybody. So keep in mind that all the stretches on the following pages do indeed stretch the iliotibial band – it's up to you to tinker around and find the one that works the best.

Step 1: Stand with your arms at your side.

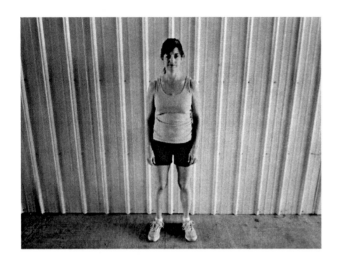

Stretch #1

Step 2: Cross your painful leg behind you. The right iliotibial band is going to be stretched in the picture below.

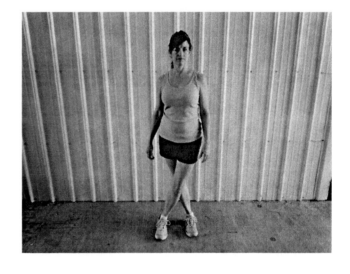

Step 3: Now put your hand on your waist and gently lean over until you feel a good stretch on the side of your leg. Hold the stretch for 15 seconds. Do three times a day.

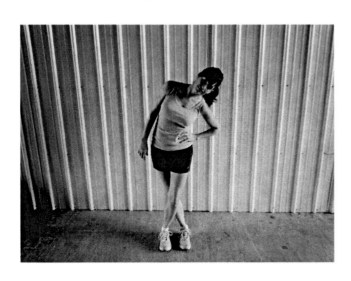

Stretch #2 is done in the same position as Stretch #1.

Stretch #2

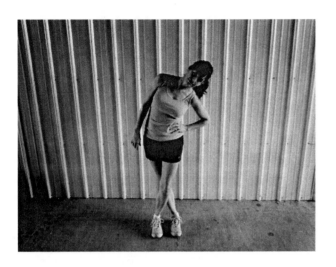

Except this time, you're going to be next to a wall.   Use the wall to help push yourself into the side-leaning position to get a stronger stretch.

Any stable object will do. Remember, hold the stretch for 15 seconds. Do three times a day.

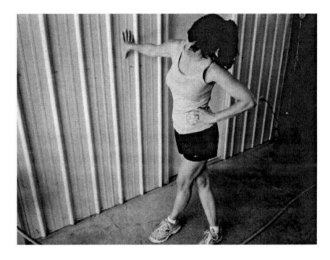

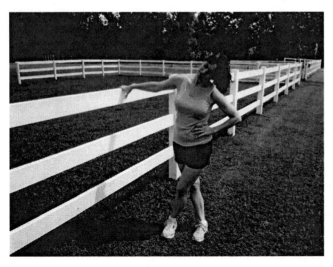

Step 1: Stand with your arms at your side.

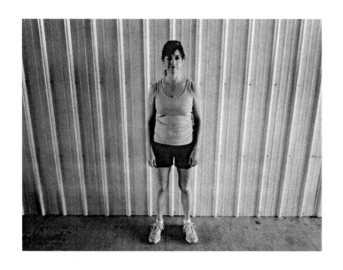

Stretch #3

Step 2: Cross your painful leg behind you. The right iliotibial band is going to be stretched in the picture below.

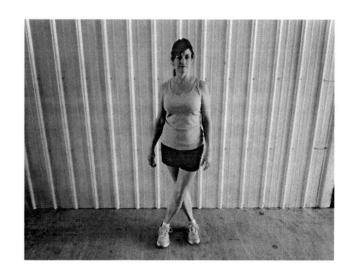

Step 3: Now bring your arm up and over your head and lean over until you feel a good stretch on the side of your leg. Hold the stretch for 15 seconds. Do three times a day.

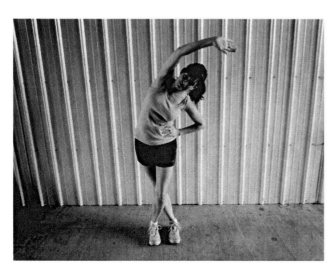

Step 1: Stand with your arms at your side.

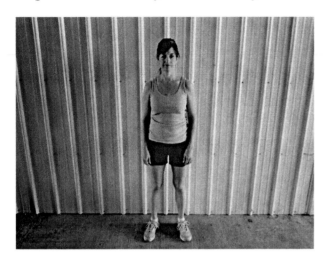

Stretch #4

Step 2: Cross your painful leg behind you. The right iliotibial band is going to be stretched in the picture below.

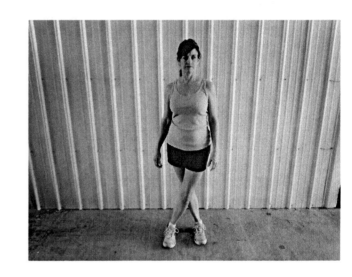

Step 3: Now bring both arms up and over your head, put your hands together, and lean over until you feel a good stretch on the side of your leg. This is a little stronger stretch than Stretch #3, because both arms are being used to stretch. Hold the stretch for 15 seconds. Do three times a day.

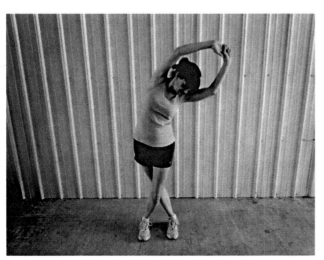

Step 1: Stand with your arms at your side.

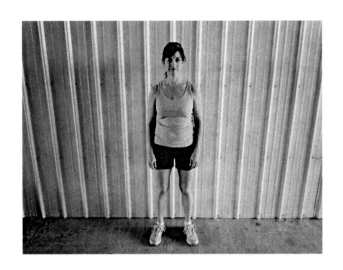

Stretch #5

Step 2: Cross your painful leg behind you. The right iliotibial band is going to be stretched in the picture below.

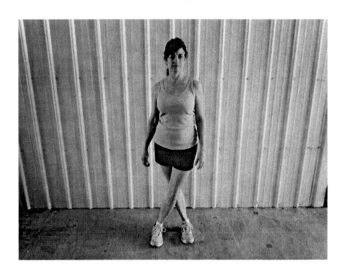

Step 3: Now bring both arms up and over your head, put your hands together, and lean over at an angle until you feel a good stretch on the side of your leg.

This stretch differs from Stretch #4, because you are leaning forward and to the side . Hold the stretch for 15 seconds. Do three times a day.

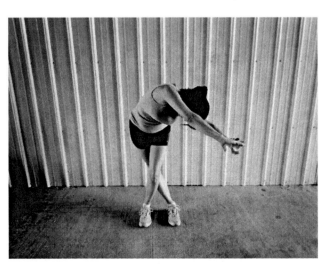

Key Points

✓ **a tightness in the iliotibial band and the muscles that connect to it could contribute to the compression that irritates the knee in iliotibial band syndrome**

✓ **some studies have shown that people with iliotibial band syndrome are tighter in their hip than pain-free controls**

✓ **many studies have included stretching as part of a treatment program for iliotibial band syndrome and have gotten good results**

✓ **stretching takes only a few minutes each day to do**

Putting It All Together

Up to this point in the book, we've built a good foundation of knowledge for you to be able to treat your own iliotibial band syndrome. With that accomplished, it's now time to put it all together in a six-week program.

Why six-weeks? Well, that's the amount of time it takes iliotibial band syndrome patients to fully recover in most studies. Here are a few key rules to always keep in mind before you begin …

- always check with your doctor before beginning an exercise program.

- the number one rule is "Do no harm." You should not be in a lot of pain while doing these exercises. Some discomfort is okay - remember that you're probably working muscles and joints you haven't used in a while, at least in this manner.

- stop the exercises if you have any significant increase in pain or symptoms. If done correctly, the exercises in this book do not put you in unsafe positions, nor do they involve any heavy weights. *However*, it's your body and your responsibility, so stop if you feel like any harm is being done.

DO THIS ON MONDAY, WEDNESDAY, and FRIDAY

Pick One of These Stretching Exercises Hold for 15 sec. 3 x day	**Two Strengthening Exercises** Do one time a day. Work up to 12 times.	**Ice Massage** 5 minutes 2 x day

Page 37 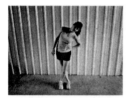   Page 27 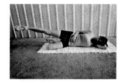   Page 20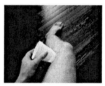

Page 38 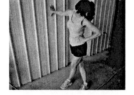   Page 30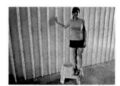

Page 39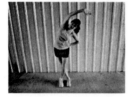

Page 40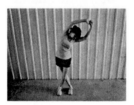

Page 41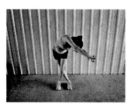

DO THESE EXERCISES ON TUESDAY, and THURSDAY

**Pick One of These
Stretching Exercises**
Hold for 15 sec.
3 x day

Ice Massage
5 minutes
2 x day

Page 37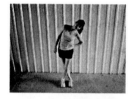

Page 20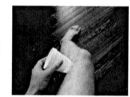

Page 38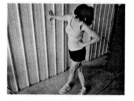

Page 39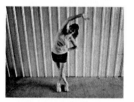

Page 40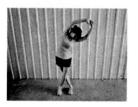

Page 41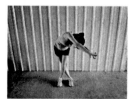

Track Your Progress!

Since it can be hard to remember from one session to the next things like how much weight you've used, it's helpful to quickly jot down this information. I've also found that when patients keep track of their exercises, it helps keep them on track too! The following is an example of how to record your progress by using the exercise sheets provided in this book...

Week 1: Monday

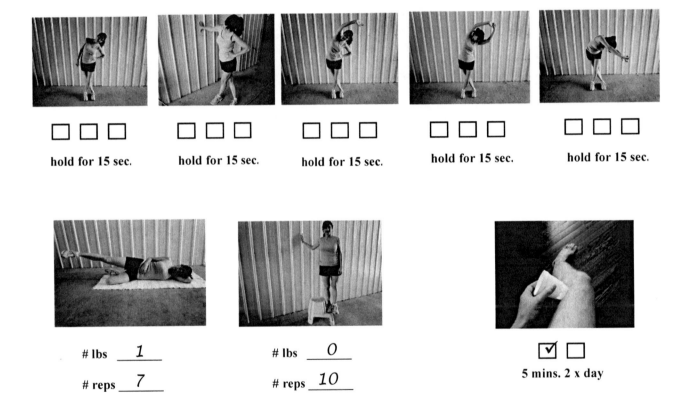

hold for 15 sec.   hold for 15 sec.   hold for 15 sec.   hold for 15 sec.   hold for 15 sec.

\# lbs _1_   \# lbs _0_

\# reps _7_   \# reps _10_   5 mins. 2 x day

Using the exercise sheets provided is easy. Starting with the group of five stretches across the top, *you only have to do one – the one that feels like it gives you the best stretch.* There are three boxes under each stretch, just check off each one after you do it.

Below the stretches are the two gluteus medius strengthening exercises - with spaces for you to write down how many reps (times) you did each exercise, and what pound ankle weight you used (if any). And lastly, to the bottom far right, are two boxes for you to check off after you perform the ice massage.

When Do I Stop?

I recommend that you do the full program for six weeks. Studies have shown that this is a sufficient amount of time for you to become pain free. If your leg feels great after six weeks, and you feel like you're where you want to be, I recommend you continue stretching your iliotibial band at least several times a week, and perform the strengthening exercises as least once a week - in order to *maintain* the progress you've made and keep you out of further trouble.

On the other hand, if you have good pain relief after doing the program for six weeks, but you're still not quite where you want to be, continue with the program until you either reach your goal, or no further progress is being made. And, if you have not seen a lick of progress after doing the program in this book for three months, then it is not a good solution for your iliotibial band syndrome.

A Word About Other Activities

I highly recommend that you discontinue running or any other activities that continue to cause pain. On the other hand, activities that *do not* provoke pain while doing them (or after doing them) are allowed as you are healing.

So when can you go back to activities that stress the iliotibial band, such as running? My general rule of thumb is that when you're a) pain free with all daily activities, and b) have been able to add a pound or two to the strengthening exercises and can do them without pain – it's okay to *ease* back into previously aggravating activities. For instance if you're a runner, try running *every other* day at first, testing out short distances. Over the next 3 to 4 weeks, try gradually increasing the distance and frequency of running.

The pages that follow contain exercise sheets for six weeks of workouts. Make additional copies as needed.

Week 1: Monday

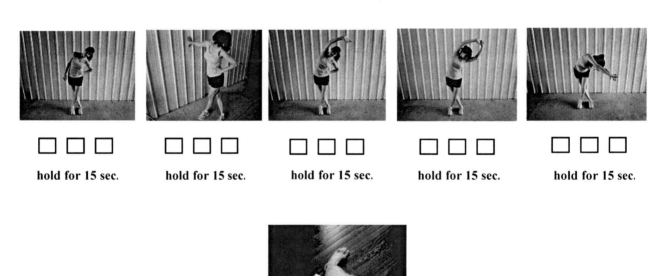

☐ ☐ ☐

hold for 15 sec.

☐ ☐ ☐

hold for 15 sec.

☐ ☐ ☐

hold for 15 sec.

☐ ☐ ☐

hold for 15 sec.

☐ ☐ ☐

hold for 15 sec.

lbs _____

reps _____

lbs _____

reps _____

☐ ☐

5 mins. 2 x day

Week 1: Tuesday

☐ ☐ ☐

hold for 15 sec.

☐ ☐ ☐

hold for 15 sec.

☐ ☐ ☐

hold for 15 sec.

☐ ☐ ☐

hold for 15 sec.

☐ ☐ ☐

hold for 15 sec.

☐ ☐

5 mins. 2 x day

Week 1: Wednesday

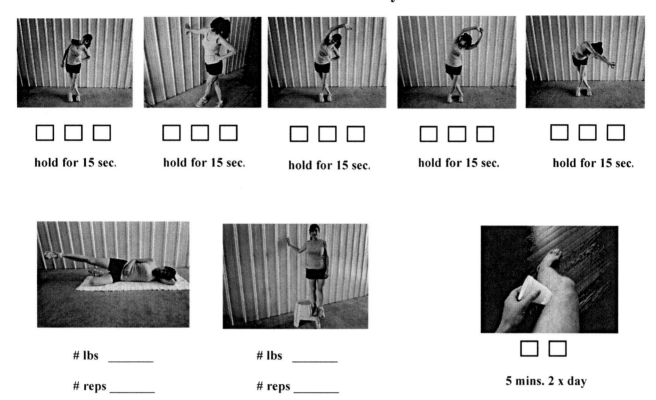

hold for 15 sec.　　hold for 15 sec.　　hold for 15 sec.　　hold for 15 sec.　　hold for 15 sec.

lbs _____　　# lbs _____

reps _____　　# reps _____

5 mins. 2 x day

Week 1: Thursday

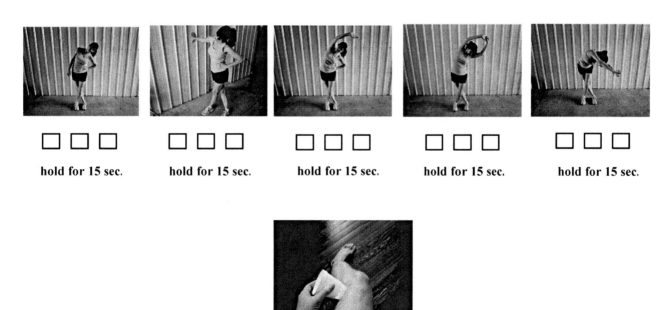

hold for 15 sec.　　hold for 15 sec.　　hold for 15 sec.　　hold for 15 sec.　　hold for 15 sec.

5 mins. 2 x day

Week 1: Friday

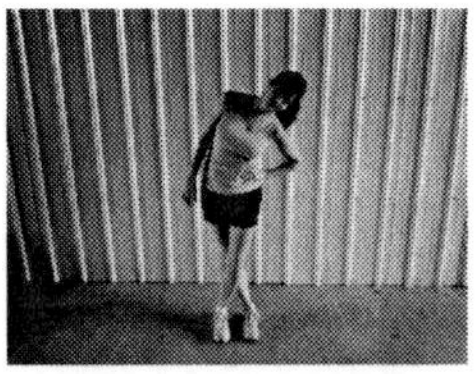

☐ ☐ ☐

hold for 15 sec.

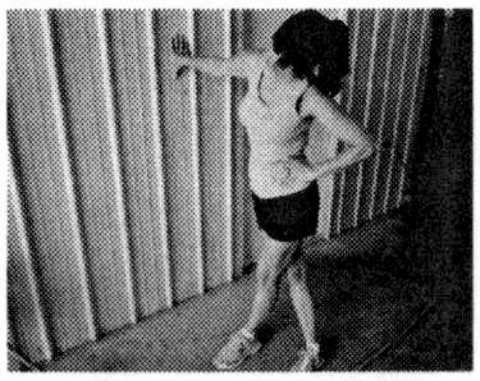

☐ ☐ ☐

hold for 15 sec.

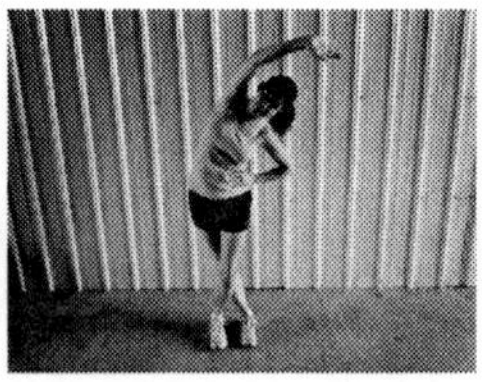

☐ ☐ ☐

hold for 15 sec.

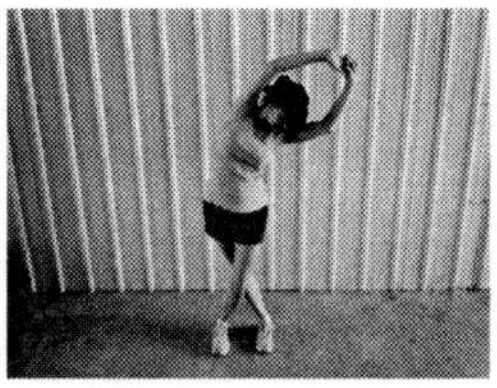

☐ ☐ ☐

hold for 15 sec.

☐ ☐ ☐

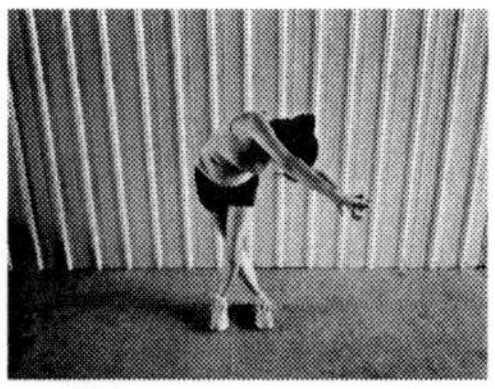

hold for 15 sec.

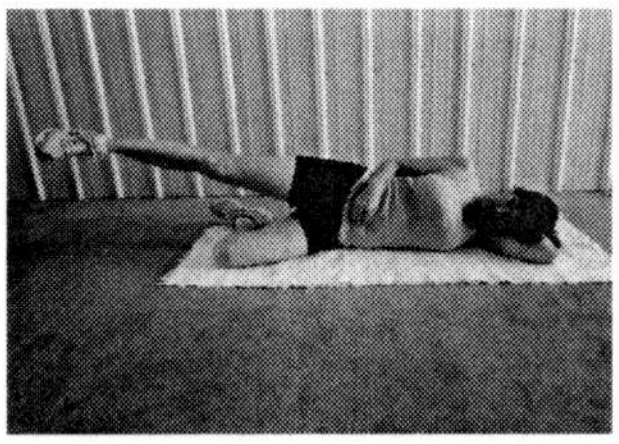

 # lbs _____

 # reps _____

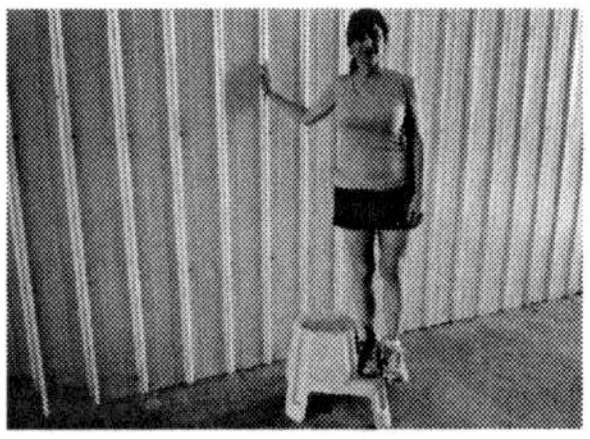

 # lbs _____

 # reps _____

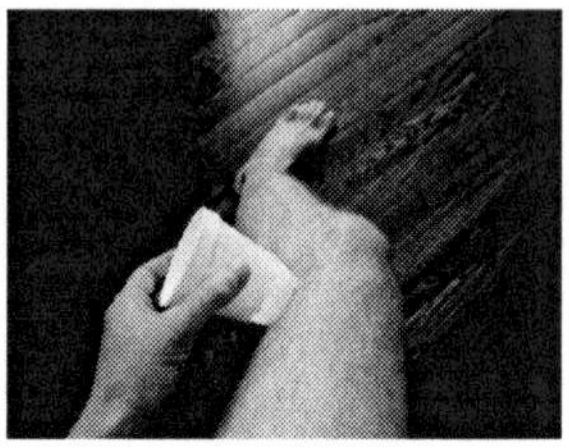

☐ ☐

5 mins. 2 x day

Week 2: Monday

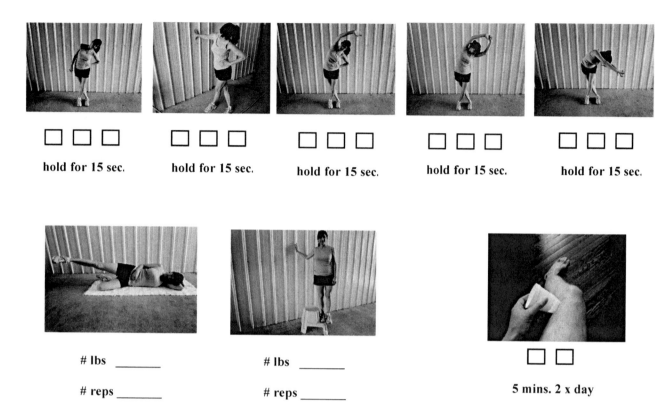

□ □ □   □ □ □   □ □ □   □ □ □   □ □ □

hold for 15 sec.   hold for 15 sec.   hold for 15 sec.   hold for 15 sec.   hold for 15 sec.

lbs _____   # lbs _____

reps _____   # reps _____

□ □

5 mins. 2 x day

Week 2: Tuesday

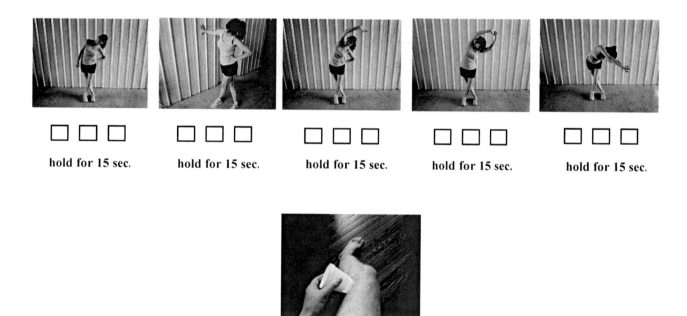

□ □ □   □ □ □   □ □ □   □ □ □   □ □ □

hold for 15 sec.   hold for 15 sec.   hold for 15 sec.   hold for 15 sec.   hold for 15 sec.

□ □

5 mins. 2 x day

Week 2: Wednesday

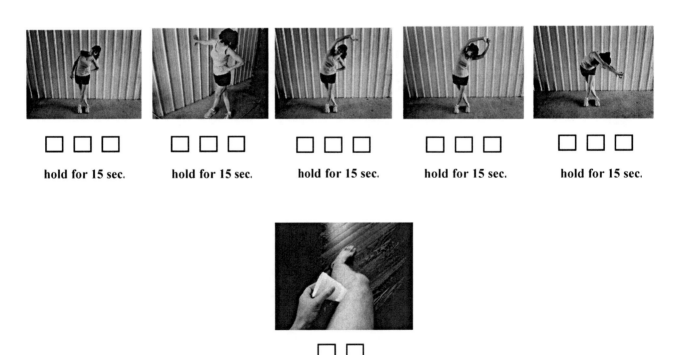

☐ ☐ ☐

hold for 15 sec.

☐ ☐ ☐

hold for 15 sec.

☐ ☐ ☐

hold for 15 sec.

☐ ☐ ☐

hold for 15 sec.

☐ ☐ ☐

hold for 15 sec.

lbs _____

reps _____

lbs _____

reps _____

☐ ☐

5 mins. 2 x day

Week 2: Thursday

☐ ☐ ☐

hold for 15 sec.

☐ ☐ ☐

hold for 15 sec.

☐ ☐ ☐

hold for 15 sec.

☐ ☐ ☐

hold for 15 sec.

☐ ☐ ☐

hold for 15 sec.

☐ ☐

5 mins. 2 x day

Week 2: Friday

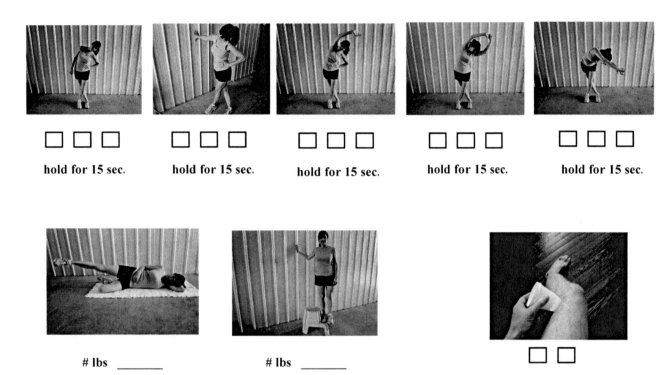

hold for 15 sec. hold for 15 sec. hold for 15 sec. hold for 15 sec. hold for 15 sec.

lbs _____

reps _____

lbs _____

reps _____

5 mins. 2 x day

Week 3: Monday

☐ ☐ ☐
hold for 15 sec.

☐ ☐ ☐
hold for 15 sec.

☐ ☐ ☐
hold for 15 sec.

☐ ☐ ☐
hold for 15 sec.

☐ ☐ ☐
hold for 15 sec.

lbs _____

reps _____

lbs _____

reps _____

☐ ☐
5 mins. 2 x day

Week 3: Tuesday

☐ ☐ ☐
hold for 15 sec.

☐ ☐ ☐
hold for 15 sec.

☐ ☐ ☐
hold for 15 sec.

☐ ☐ ☐
hold for 15 sec.

☐ ☐ ☐
hold for 15 sec.

☐ ☐
5 mins. 2 x day

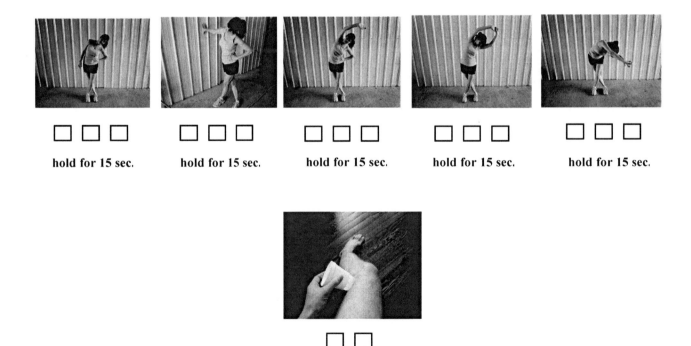

Week 3: Wednesday

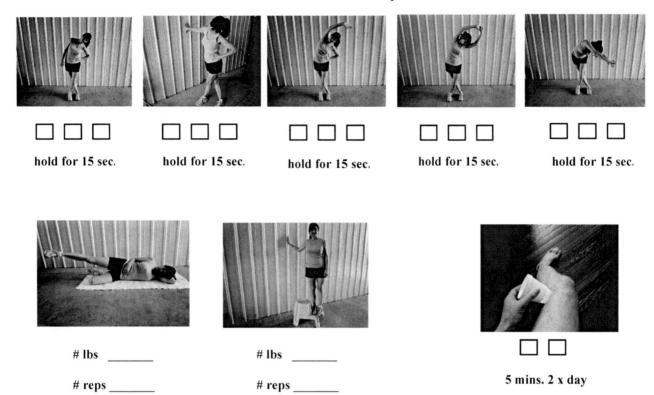

☐ ☐ ☐

hold for 15 sec.

☐ ☐ ☐

hold for 15 sec.

☐ ☐ ☐

hold for 15 sec.

☐ ☐ ☐

hold for 15 sec.

☐ ☐ ☐

hold for 15 sec.

lbs _____

reps _____

lbs _____

reps _____

☐ ☐

5 mins. 2 x day

Week 3: Thursday

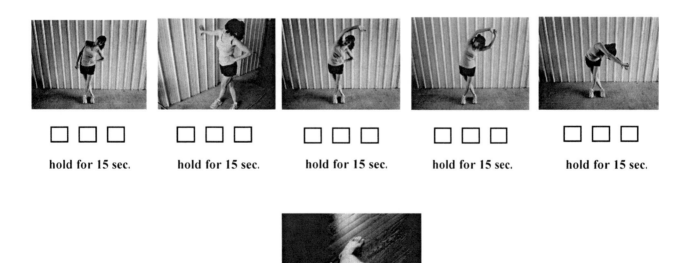

☐ ☐ ☐

hold for 15 sec.

☐ ☐ ☐

hold for 15 sec.

☐ ☐ ☐

hold for 15 sec.

☐ ☐ ☐

hold for 15 sec.

☐ ☐ ☐

hold for 15 sec.

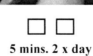

☐ ☐

5 mins. 2 x day

Week 3: Friday

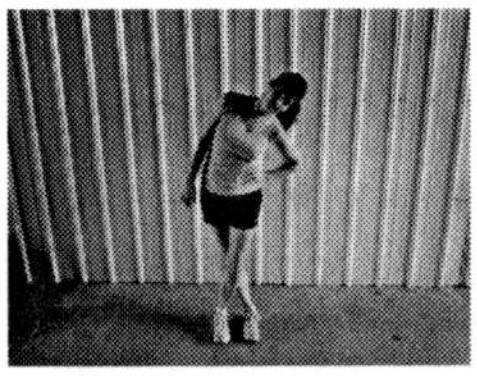

☐ ☐ ☐

hold for 15 sec.

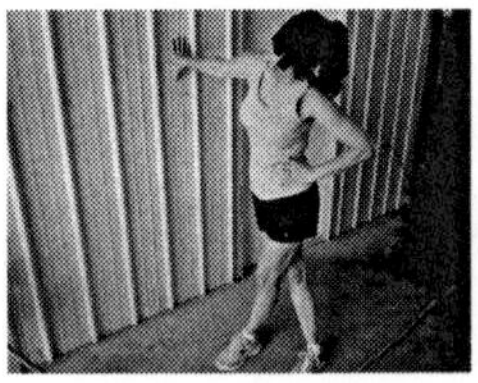

☐ ☐ ☐

hold for 15 sec.

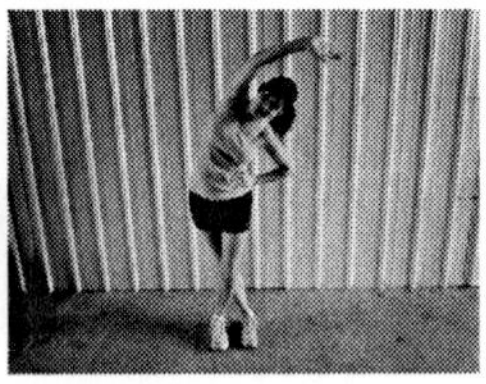

☐ ☐ ☐

hold for 15 sec.

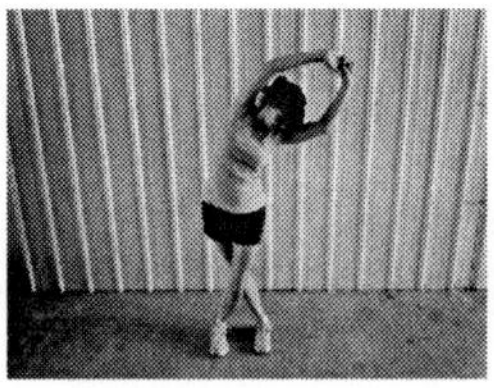

☐ ☐ ☐

hold for 15 sec.

☐ ☐ ☐

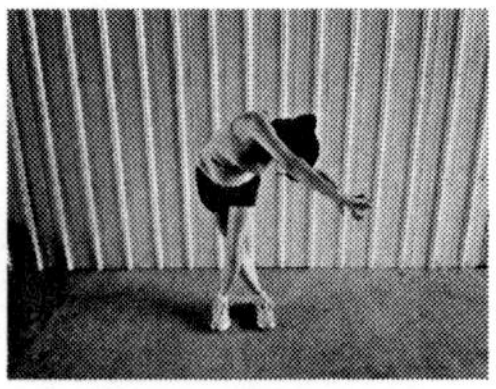

hold for 15 sec.

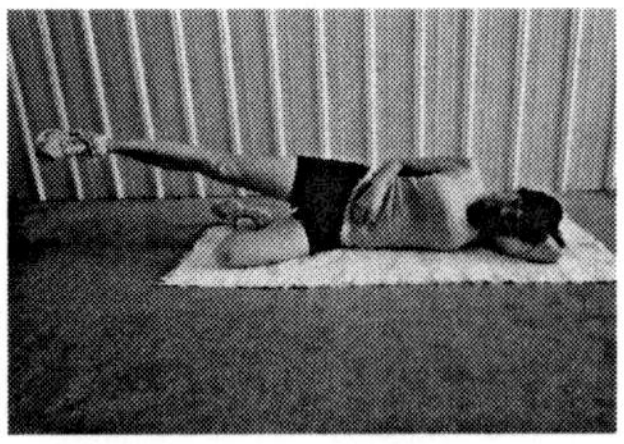

lbs _____

reps _____

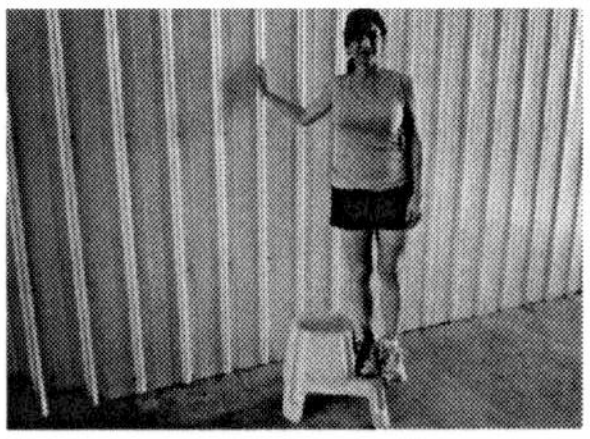

lbs _____

reps _____

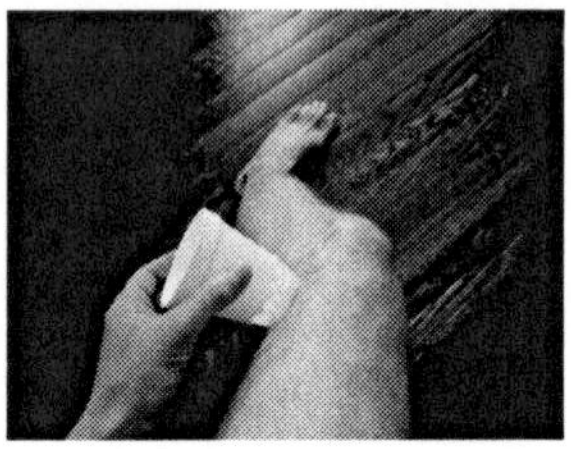

☐ ☐

5 mins. 2 x day

Week 4: Monday

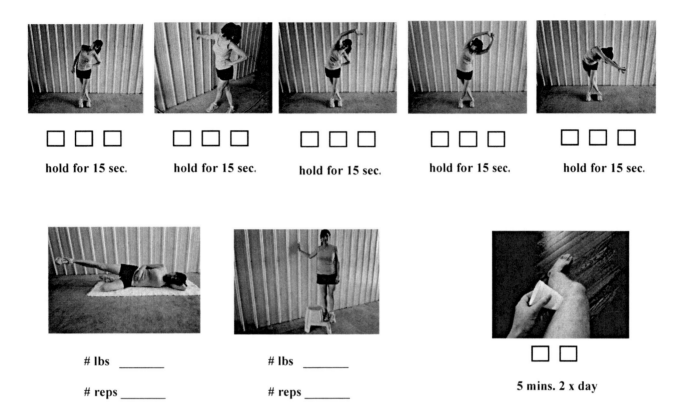

□ □ □   □ □ □   □ □ □   □ □ □   □ □ □

hold for 15 sec.   hold for 15 sec.   hold for 15 sec.   hold for 15 sec.   hold for 15 sec.

lbs _____   # lbs _____

reps _____   # reps _____

□ □

5 mins. 2 x day

Week 4: Tuesday

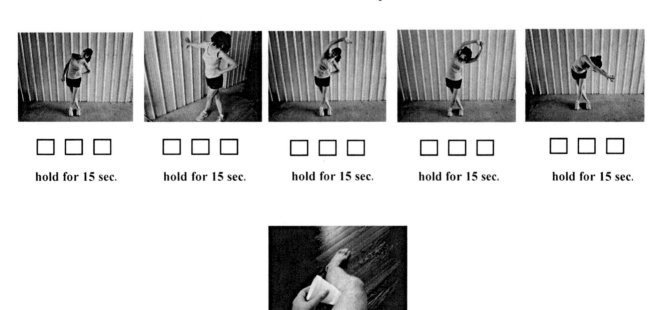

□ □ □   □ □ □   □ □ □   □ □ □   □ □ □

hold for 15 sec.   hold for 15 sec.   hold for 15 sec.   hold for 15 sec.   hold for 15 sec.

□ □

5 mins. 2 x day

Week 4: Wednesday

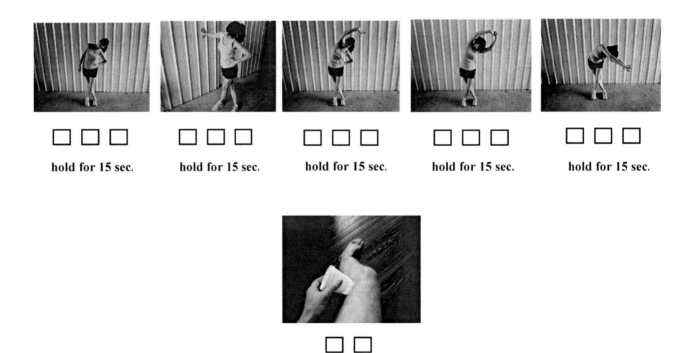

☐ ☐ ☐	☐ ☐ ☐	☐ ☐ ☐	☐ ☐ ☐	☐ ☐ ☐
hold for 15 sec.	hold for 15 sec.	hold for 15 sec.	hold for 15 sec.	hold for 15 sec.

# lbs _____	# lbs _____	
# reps _____	# reps _____	☐ ☐
		5 mins. 2 x day

Week 4: Thursday

☐ ☐ ☐	☐ ☐ ☐	☐ ☐ ☐	☐ ☐ ☐	☐ ☐ ☐
hold for 15 sec.	hold for 15 sec.	hold for 15 sec.	hold for 15 sec.	hold for 15 sec.

☐ ☐

5 mins. 2 x day

Week 4: Friday

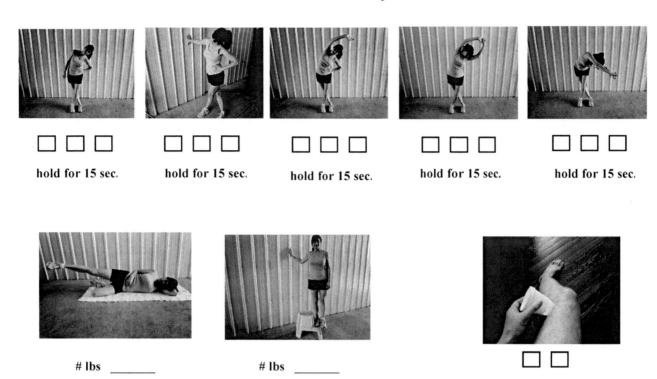

| hold for 15 sec. | hold for 15 sec. | hold for 15 sec. | hold for 15 sec. | hold for 15 sec. |

lbs _____

reps _____

lbs _____

reps _____

5 mins. 2 x day

Week 5: Monday

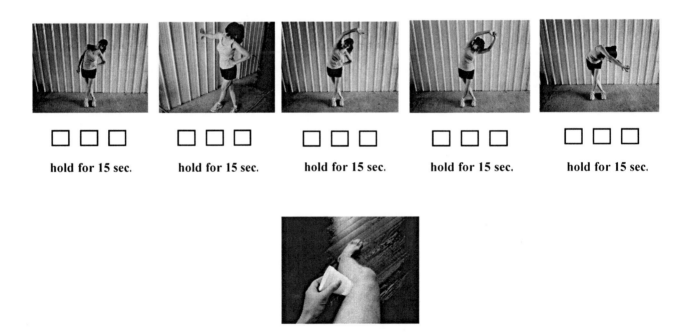

☐ ☐ ☐
hold for 15 sec.

☐ ☐ ☐
hold for 15 sec.

☐ ☐ ☐
hold for 15 sec.

☐ ☐ ☐
hold for 15 sec.

☐ ☐ ☐
hold for 15 sec.

lbs _____

reps _____

lbs _____

reps _____

☐ ☐
5 mins. 2 x day

Week 5: Tuesday

☐ ☐ ☐
hold for 15 sec.

☐ ☐ ☐
hold for 15 sec.

☐ ☐ ☐
hold for 15 sec.

☐ ☐ ☐
hold for 15 sec.

☐ ☐ ☐
hold for 15 sec.

☐ ☐
5 mins. 2 x day

Week 5: Wednesday

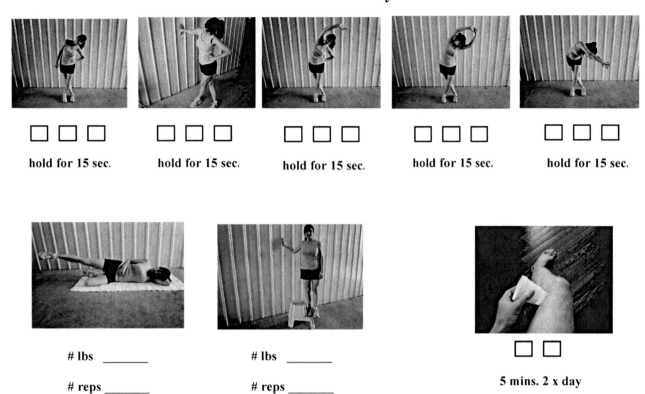

□ □ □	□ □ □	□ □ □	□ □ □	□ □ □
hold for 15 sec.	hold for 15 sec.	hold for 15 sec.	hold for 15 sec.	hold for 15 sec.

lbs _____

reps _____

lbs _____

reps _____

□ □

5 mins. 2 x day

Week 5: Thursday

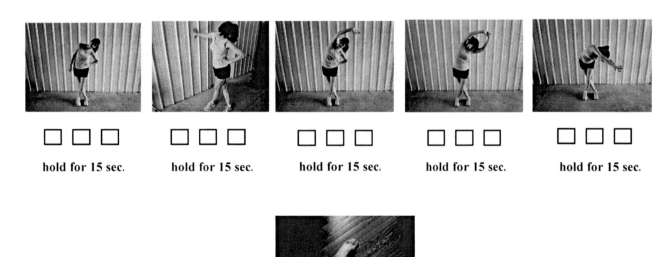

□ □ □	□ □ □	□ □ □	□ □ □	□ □ □
hold for 15 sec.	hold for 15 sec.	hold for 15 sec.	hold for 15 sec.	hold for 15 sec.

□ □

5 mins. 2 x day

Week 5: Friday

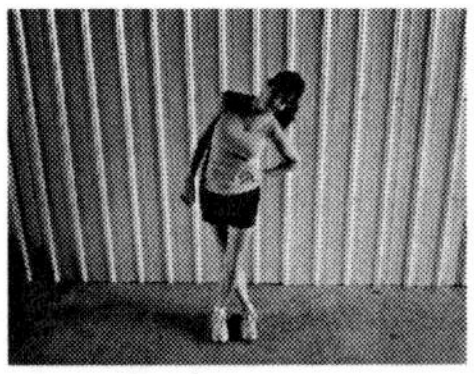

☐ ☐ ☐

hold for 15 sec.

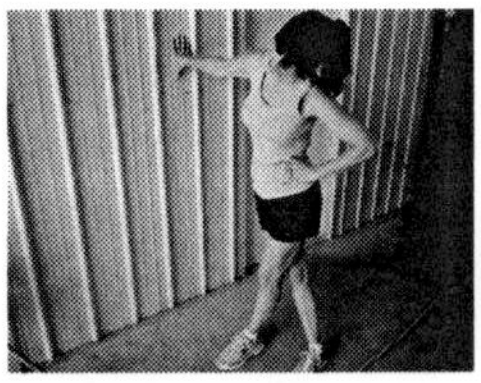

☐ ☐ ☐

hold for 15 sec.

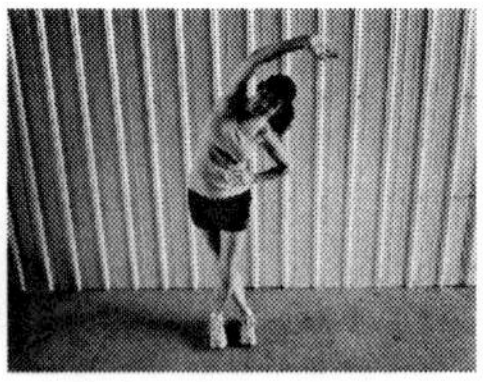

☐ ☐ ☐

hold for 15 sec.

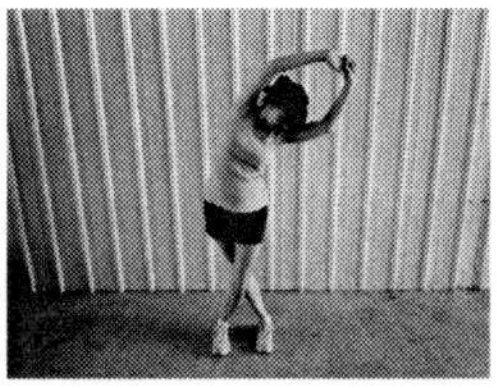

☐ ☐ ☐

hold for 15 sec.

☐ ☐ ☐

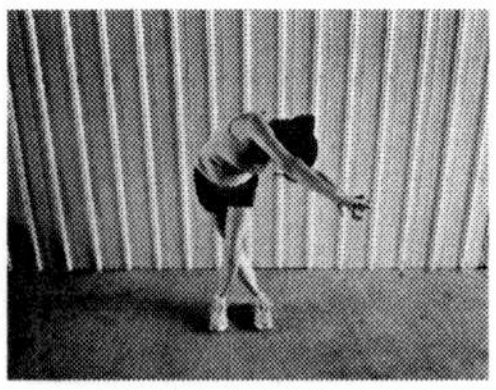

hold for 15 sec.

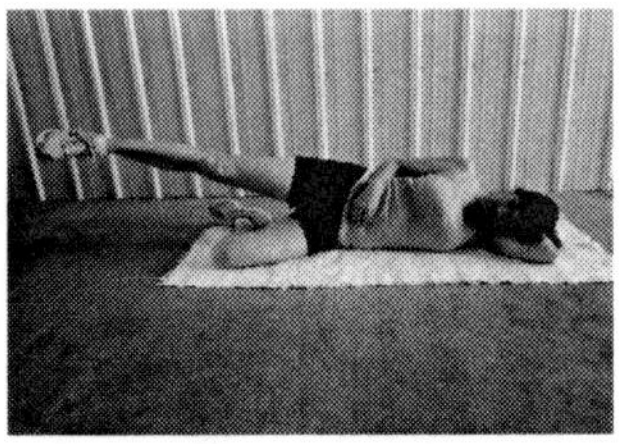

lbs _____

reps _____

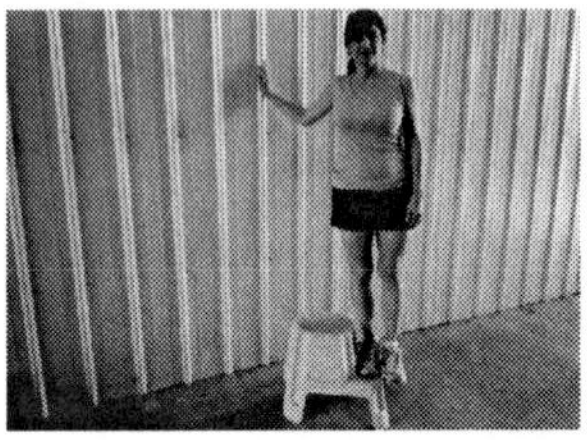

lbs _____

reps _____

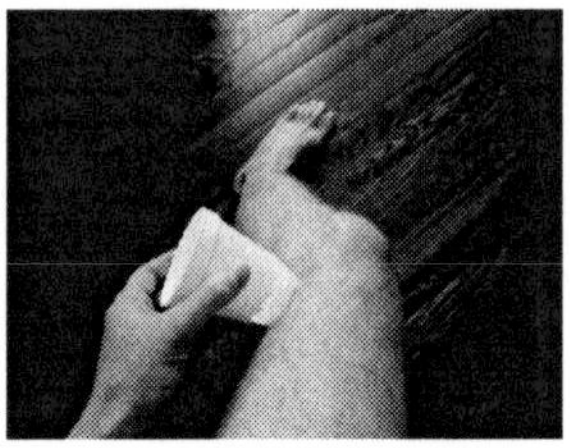

☐ ☐

5 mins. 2 x day

Week 6: Monday

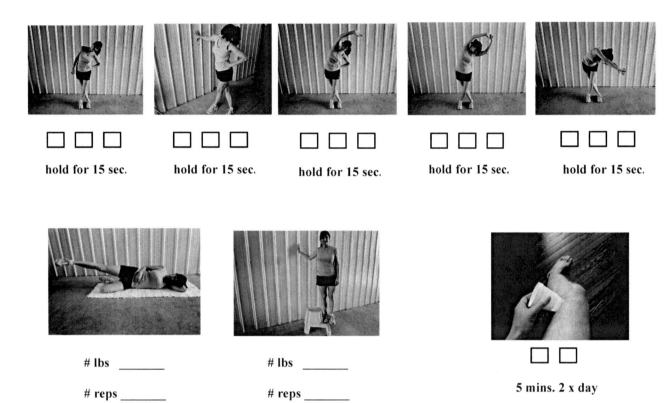

☐ ☐ ☐

hold for 15 sec.

☐ ☐ ☐

hold for 15 sec.

☐ ☐ ☐

hold for 15 sec.

☐ ☐ ☐

hold for 15 sec.

☐ ☐ ☐

hold for 15 sec.

lbs _____

reps _____

lbs _____

reps _____

☐ ☐

5 mins. 2 x day

Week 6: Tuesday

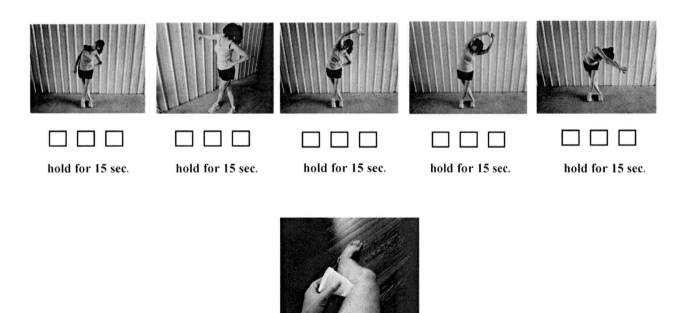

☐ ☐ ☐

hold for 15 sec.

☐ ☐ ☐

hold for 15 sec.

☐ ☐ ☐

hold for 15 sec.

☐ ☐ ☐

hold for 15 sec.

☐ ☐ ☐

hold for 15 sec.

☐ ☐

5 mins. 2 x day

Week 6: Wednesday

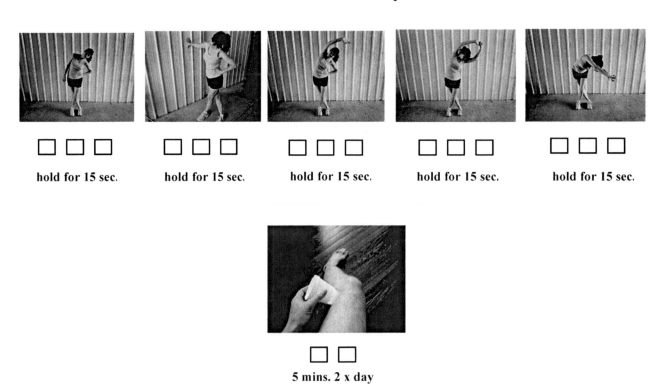

☐ ☐ ☐	☐ ☐ ☐	☐ ☐ ☐	☐ ☐ ☐	☐ ☐ ☐
hold for 15 sec.	hold for 15 sec.	hold for 15 sec.	hold for 15 sec.	hold for 15 sec.

lbs _____   # lbs _____

reps _____   # reps _____

☐ ☐

5 mins. 2 x day

Week 6: Thursday

☐ ☐ ☐	☐ ☐ ☐	☐ ☐ ☐	☐ ☐ ☐	☐ ☐ ☐
hold for 15 sec.	hold for 15 sec.	hold for 15 sec.	hold for 15 sec.	hold for 15 sec.

☐ ☐

5 mins. 2 x day

Week 6: Friday

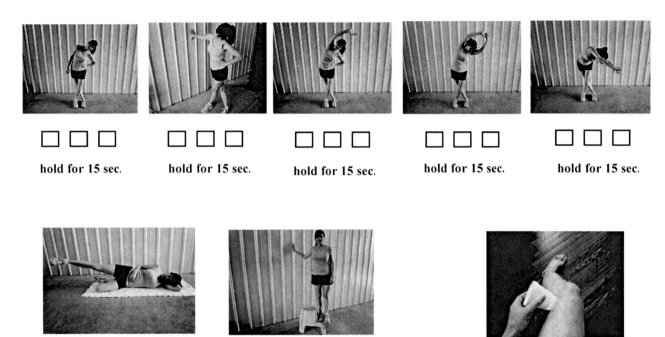

| □ □ □ | □ □ □ | □ □ □ | □ □ □ | □ □ □ |
| hold for 15 sec. | hold for 15 sec. | hold for 15 sec. | hold for 15 sec. | hold for 15 sec. |

lbs _____

reps _____

lbs _____

reps _____

□ □

5 mins. 2 x day

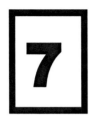

Why Measuring Your Progress Is *Very* Important

Okay. You've learned all about iliotibial band syndrome, have started the exercises, and are on the road to recovery. So now what should you expect?

Well, we all know you should expect to get better. But what exactly does *better* mean? As a physical therapist treating patients, it means two distinct things to me:

- your knee starts to *feel* better

and

- your knee starts to *work* better

And so, when a patient returns for a follow-up visit, I will re-assess them, looking for specific changes in their knee **pain**, as well as their knee **function**.

In this book, I'm going to recommend that readers do the same thing periodically. Why? Simply because people in pain can't always see the progress they're making. For instance, sometimes a person's knee pain doesn't seem to be getting any better, but they can now do some motions or tasks that they couldn't do before - a sure sign that things *are* healing. Or, sometimes a person still has significant knee pain, but they're not looking at the fact that it's actually occurring less frequently - yet another good indication that positive changes are taking place.

Whatever the case may be, if a person isn't looking at the big picture, and doesn't think they're getting any better, they're likely to get discouraged and stop doing their exercises altogether - even though they really might have been on the right track!

On the other hand though, what if you periodically check your progress and are keenly aware that your knee *is* making some changes for the better? What if you can *positively* see *objective* results? My guess is that you're going to be giving yourself a healthy dose of motivation to keep on truckin' with the exercises.

Having said that, I'm going to show you exactly what to check for from time-to-time so that you can monitor the changes that are taking place. I call them "outcomes" and there are two of them.

Outcome #1:
Look for Changes in Your Pain

First of all, you should look for changes in your pain. I know this may sound silly, but sometimes it's my job to get a person to see that their pain *is* actually improving. You see, a lot of people come to physical therapy thinking they're going to be pain-free right away. Then, when they're not instantly better and still having pain, they often start to worry and become discouraged. Truth is, I have yet to put a patient on an exercise program for iliotibial band syndrome and have them get instantly better. Better yes, but not *instantly* better.

Over the years, I have found that patients usually respond to the exercises in a quite predictable pattern. One of three things will almost always occur as patients begin to turn the corner and get better:

- your knee pain will be just as intense as always,
  however now it is occurring much less frequently

or

- your knee pain is now *less* intense, even though
  it is still occurring just as frequently

or

- you start to notice less intense knee pain *and* it is
  now occurring less frequently

The point here is to make sure that you keep a sharp eye out for any of these three changes as you progress with the exercises. If *any* of them occur, it will be a sure sign that the exercises are helping and you're on the right track. You can then look forward to the pain gradually getting better, usually over the weeks to come.

Outcome #2:
Look for Changes in Knee Function

Looking at how well your knee works is very important because many times knee function improves *before* the pain does. For example, sometimes a patient will do the exercises for a while, and although their knee will still hurt a lot, they are able to do many things that they hadn't been able to in a while – a really good indicator that healing is taking place *and* that the pain should be easing up soon.

While measuring your knee function may sound like a pain in the butt, it doesn't have to be. In this book, I'm recommending that readers use a quick and easy assessment tool known as *The Knee Injury and Osteoarthritis Outcome Score-Physical Function Short-Form* (Perruccio 2008). Well, let's just call it the KOOS-PS for short.

While the name certainly sounds like a nightmare, the KOOS-PS is a really useful tool you can use to keep track of how your knee is *functioning*. Studies show that it is a valid test (Davis 2009), has good test-retest reliability (Ornetti 2009, Goncalves 2010), and is responsive to clinical changes (Davis 2009). And best of all, *it takes only a couple of minutes to complete*. Now that's my kinda test!

So what exactly does taking the KOOS-PS involve? Not much.

- you read the instructions and then simply check the degree of difficulty you have doing each of the seven activities
- next, you add up your points and use a table to get your score

On the next page is the KOOS-PS, let's have a look….

KOOS-Physical Function Shortform (KOOS-PS)

INSTRUCTIONS: This survey asks for your view about your knee. This information will help us keep track of how well you are able to perform different activities.

Answer every question by checking the appropriate box, only one box for each question. If you are unsure about how to answer a question, please give the best answer you can so that you answer all the questions.

The following questions concern your level of function in performing usual daily activities and higher level activities. For each of the following activities, please indicate the degree of difficulty you have experienced in the **last week** due to your knee problem.

1. Rising from bed

None	Mild	Moderate	Severe	Extreme
❑	❑	❑	❑	❑

2. Putting on socks/stockings

None	Mild	Moderate	Severe	Extreme
❑	❑	❑	❑	❑

3. Rising from sitting

None	Mild	Moderate	Severe	Extreme
❑	❑	❑	❑	❑

4. Bending to floor

None	Mild	Moderate	Severe	Extreme
❑	❑	❑	❑	❑

5. Twisting/pivoting on your injured knee

None	Mild	Moderate	Severe	Extreme
❑	❑	❑	❑	❑

6. Kneeling

None	Mild	Moderate	Severe	Extreme
❑	❑	❑	❑	❑

7. Squatting

None	Mild	Moderate	Severe	Extreme
❑	❑	❑	❑	❑

your total points	your score
0	0
1	5.6
2	10.5
3	14.8
4	18.63
5	22
6	24.9
7	27.5
8	29.7
9	31.8
10	33.6
11	35.3
12	37
13	38.6
14	40.3
15	42
16	44
17	46.1
18	48.5
19	51.2
20	54.4
21	57.9
22	62
23	66.6
24	71.8
25	77.7
26	84.3
27	91.8
28	100

After you're done completing the KOOS-PS, you're going to give yourself points based on the boxes you've just checked. So…

- give yourself 1 point every time you checked "mild"
- give yourself 2 points every time you checked "moderate"
- give yourself 3 points every time you checked "severe"
- give yourself 4 points every time you checked "extreme"

Go ahead and add up the points, which will equal a number anywhere from 0 to 28.

Now, using the table on the right, take your point total number, and find it in the *left* hand column. Found it? Okay, your score will be the number that is directly to the *right* of it, in the right hand column.

For example, let's say you added up the points and your total points equaled 16. Just find the number 16 in the left hand column, and your score will be just to the right, which would be 44.

So what was your score? Keep in mind that scores will range anywhere from a 0 to a 100. Higher scores mean you're in bad shape, so your goal is to score as *low* as possible. In other words, a score of 0 means you're having *no* difficulty doing any of the activities listed in the survey, while a score of 100 means you're having a lot of trouble.

If you did score high though, don't worry. Just keep taking the KOOS-PS every few weeks, and as you progress with the exercises, you should see your score go lower and lower as time passes. Remember, sometimes knee function gets better *before* the pain does.

Quick Review

✓ being aware of your progress is an important part of treating your iliotibial band syndrome – it motivates you to keep doing the exercises.

✓ look for the pain to become less *intense*, less *frequent*, or both to let you know that the exercises are helping

✓ sometimes your knee starts to work better *before* it starts to feel better. Taking the *KOOS-PS* from time-to-time makes you aware of improving knee function

---

References

Well, we've come a long way since page one. Now that we're coming to the end, I'd like to take a few minutes to show you all the research that went into this book.

The following is a list of all the randomized controlled trials and scientific studies that have been published in peer-reviewed journals that this book is based on. To make a long story short, there's no nonsense going on here – *every* piece of information you've just read has a good evidence-based reason for being here!

Having said that, I've included this handy reference section so that readers can check out the information for themselves if they wish. Good luck!

Chapter 2

Fairclough J, et al. The functional anatomy of the iliotibial band during flexion and extension of the knee: implications for understanding iliotibial band syndrome. *J Anat* 2006;208:309-316.

Falvey E.C., et al. Iliotibial band syndrome: an examination of the evidence behind a number of treatment options. *Scand J Med Sci Sports* 2010;20:580-587.

Murphy B, et al. Iliotibial band friction syndrome: MR imaging findings. *Radiology* 1992;185:569-571.

Muhle C, et al. Iliotibial band friction syndrome: MR imaging findings in 16 patients and MR arthrographic study of six cadaveric knees. *Radiology* 1999;212:103-110.

Nemeth W, et al. The lateral synovial recess of the knee: anatomy and role in chronic iliotibial band friction syndrome. *Arthroscopy* 1996;12:574-580.

Nishimura G, et al. MR findings in iliotibial band syndrome. *Skeletal Radiology* 1997;26:533-537.

Noble C. Iliotibial band friction syndrome in runners. *The American Journal of Sports Medicine* 1980;8:232-234.

Chapter 3

Gunter P, et al. Local corticosteroid injection in iliotibial band friction syndrome in runners: a randomized controlled trial. *Br J Sports Med* 2004;38:269-272.

Lowden B, et al. Determinants and nature of intramuscular temperature changes during cold therapy. *Am J Phys Med* 1975;54:223-233.

Zemke J, et al. Intramuscular temperature responses in the human leg to two forms of cryotherapy: ice massage and ice bag. *Journal of Orthopaedic and Sports Physical Therapy* 1998;4:301-307.

Chapter 4

Beers A, et al. Effects of multi-modal physiotherapy, including hip abductor strengthening, in patients with iliotibial band friction syndrome. *Physiother Can* 2008;60:180-188.

Fredericson M, et al. Hip abductor weakness in distance runners with iliotibial band syndrome. *Clinical Journal of Sports Medicine* 2000;10:169-175.

Niemuth P, et al. Hip muscle weakness and overuse injuries in recreational runners. *Clin J Sports Med* 2005;15:14-21.

Chapter 5

Beers A, et al. Effects of multi-modal physiotherapy, including hip abductor strengthening, in patients with iliotibial band friction syndrome. *Physiother Can* 2008;60:180-188.

Fredericson M, et al. Hip abductor weakness in distance runners with iliotibial band syndrome. *Clinical Journal of Sports Medicine* 2000;10:169-175.

Grau S, et al. Kinematic classification of iliotibial band syndrome in runners. *Scan J Med Sci Sports* 2011;21:184-189.

Schwellnus M.P., et al. Anti-inflammatory and combined anti-inflammatory/analgesic medication in the early management of iliotibial band friction syndrome. A clinical trial. *S Afr Med J* 1991;79:602-606.

Chapter 7

Davis A, et al. Comparative, validity and responsiveness of the HOOS-PS and KOOS-PS to the WOMAC physical function subscale in total joint replacement for osteoarthritis. *Osteoarthritis and Cartilage* 2009;17:843-847.

Goncalves R, et al. Reliability, validity and responsiveness of the Portuguese version of the knee injury and osteoarthritis outcome score-physical function short-form (KOOS-PS). Osteoarthritis and Cartilage 2010;18:372-376.

Ornetti P, et al. Psychometric properties of the French translation of the reduced KOOS and HOOS (KOOS-PS and HOOS-PS) *Osteoarthritis and Cartilage* 2009;17:1604-1608.

Perruccio A, et al. The development of a short measure of physical function for knee OA KOOS-Physical function shortform (KOOS-PS)- an OARSI/OMERACT initiative. *Osteoarthritis and Cartilage* 2008;16:542-550.